The Power of Intermittent Fasting for Women

"Achieving Optimal Health and Fitness"

PETER MILLER

Introduction

Intermittent fasting has become a popular approach to eating in recent years, with many people using it as a way to improve their overall health and wellbeing. This eating strategy involves alternating periods of fasting with periods of eating, and it has been shown to have numerous benefits, including weight loss, improved blood sugar control, and reduced inflammation.

While intermittent fasting can be effective for both men and women, there are specific considerations that women need to take into account when adopting this approach to eating. Women have different hormonal profiles and nutritional needs than men, and these differences can impact how they respond to intermittent fasting. As a result, women may need to modify their approach to intermittent fasting to achieve optimal health and fitness.

In this book, we will explore the benefits of intermittent fasting for women and why they need a different approach to this eating strategy. We will also provide practical tips and strategies for women who want to try intermittent fasting, as well as address common concerns that women may have about fasting.

The Benefits of Intermittent Fasting for Women:

Intermittent fasting has been shown to have numerous benefits for both men and women, including weight loss, improved insulin sensitivity, and reduced inflammation. However, women may also experience specific benefits from intermittent fasting due to their unique hormonal profile.

One of the most significant benefits of intermittent fasting for women is improved hormone balance. Hormones play a critical role in many aspects of women's health, including menstrual cycles, fertility, and menopause. When hormone levels are imbalanced, women may experience a range of symptoms, including mood swings, weight gain, and fatigue.

Intermittent fasting has been shown to improve hormone balance in women by reducing insulin levels and increasing growth hormone production. This can lead to better blood sugar control, reduced inflammation, and improved metabolic health. Women who fast may also experience a reduction in menstrual symptoms, such as cramps and bloating.

Another benefit of intermittent fasting for women is increased energy and mental clarity. When the body is in a fasted state, it shifts from using glucose for energy to using stored fat. This can lead to increased energy levels and improved mental clarity. Women who fast may also experience improved sleep quality, as the body produces more melatonin during periods of fasting.

Intermittent fasting can also be an effective strategy for weight loss and weight management in women. By restricting the times when food is consumed, women may naturally consume fewer calories overall. Additionally, intermittent fasting has been shown to increase metabolism and improve fat burning, which can lead to greater weight loss over time.

Why Women Need a Different Approach to Intermittent Fasting:

While intermittent fasting can be effective for both men and women, women need to take a different approach to fasting due to their unique hormonal profile and nutritional needs. Women have lower levels of testosterone than men, which means that they may have a harder time building and maintaining muscle mass.

Additionally, women require more nutrients than men, such as iron and folate, due to their reproductive system. Women who fast may be at risk of nutrient deficiencies, which can impact their overall health and wellbeing.

Women also have different considerations when it comes to fasting and their menstrual cycle. While fasting may help to reduce menstrual symptoms, women who fast may also experience irregular periods or missed periods. Additionally, women who are pregnant or breastfeeding should not fast, as it can impact the health of the baby.

In order for women to achieve optimal health and fitness through intermittent fasting, they need to modify their approach to suit their unique needs. This may involve adjusting the length of fasting periods, incorporating nutrient-dense foods into their diet, and taking supplements to support their health.

Conclusion:

Intermittent fasting can be a powerful tool for improving health and fitness in women, but it requires a different approach than for men. Women need to consider their unique hormonal profile and nutritional needs when adopting intermittent fasting. By doing so, women can reap the many benefits of this eating strategy while minimizing any potential risks or negative impacts on their health.

Throughout this book, we will explore the specific strategies and considerations that women need to take into account when adopting intermittent fasting. We will provide practical tips and advice for getting started with intermittent fasting, including guidance on adjusting fasting periods, incorporating nutrient-dense foods into your diet, and addressing common concerns that women may have about fasting.

Ultimately, our goal is to empower women to take control of their health and wellbeing through intermittent fasting. By adopting a thoughtful and intentional approach to fasting, women can achieve optimal health and fitness, improve their hormonal balance, and feel their best. We hope that this book will serve as a valuable resource for women who are interested in exploring the power of intermittent fasting for their own health and wellness.

Chapter 1

Understanding Intermittent Fasting

Intermittent fasting has become a popular approach to eating in recent years, with many people using it as a way to improve their health and achieve their fitness goals. In this chapter, we will explore what intermittent fasting is, the different types of intermittent fasting, and how it works to improve health and wellbeing.

What is Intermittent Fasting?

Intermittent fasting is an eating strategy that involves alternating periods of fasting with periods of eating. During the fasting period, no calories are consumed, while during the eating period, normal caloric intake is maintained.

There are many different ways to approach intermittent fasting, and the length and frequency of fasting periods can vary. Some people choose to fast for a set number of hours each day, while others may fast for entire days or multiple days in a row. The goal of intermittent fasting is to create a calorie deficit and induce a state of ketosis, in which the body burns fat for fuel instead of glucose.

The Different Types of Intermittent Fasting

There are several different types of intermittent fasting, each with its own set of guidelines and protocols. Here are some of the most common types of intermittent fasting:

- Time-restricted feeding: This type of intermittent fasting involves restricting your eating window to a certain number of hours each day, typically between 8 and 10 hours. During the fasting period, no calories are consumed, while during the eating period, normal caloric intake is maintained.

- Alternate-day fasting: This type of intermittent fasting involves alternating between days of normal eating and days of fasting. During the fasting days, no calories are consumed, while during the eating days, normal caloric intake is maintained.

- 5:2 fasting: This type of intermittent fasting involves eating normally for five days of the week and restricting calories to 500-600 calories on two non-consecutive days of the week.

- Eat-stop-eat: This type of intermittent fasting involves fasting for 24 hours, once or twice a week.

- Warrior diet: This type of intermittent fasting involves eating one large meal per day, typically in the evening, and fasting during the rest of the day.

How Intermittent Fasting Works

Intermittent fasting works by creating a calorie deficit, which in turn leads to weight loss and improved health markers. When the body is in a fasted state, it shifts from using glucose for energy to using stored fat. This can lead to increased fat burning and improved metabolic health.

Intermittent fasting has also been shown to improve insulin sensitivity, reduce inflammation, and promote autophagy, a process in which the body breaks down and recycles old or damaged cells. This can help to reduce the risk of chronic diseases such as diabetes, heart disease, and cancer.

Additionally, intermittent fasting can help to regulate hormone levels and improve hormone balance. During periods of fasting, the body produces more growth hormone, which can improve muscle growth and repair. Fasting can also help to reduce insulin levels, which can lead to better blood sugar control and reduced inflammation.

Overall, intermittent fasting is a powerful tool for improving health and wellbeing. By creating a calorie deficit and inducing a state of ketosis, intermittent fasting can lead to weight loss, improved metabolic health, and reduced risk of chronic diseases.

Chapter 2

The Benefits of Intermittent Fasting for Women

Intermittent fasting is a powerful tool for improving health and wellbeing in both men and women. However, women may experience unique benefits from this eating strategy due to their unique hormonal profile and nutritional needs. In this chapter, we will explore the many benefits of intermittent fasting for women, including improved hormone balance, increased energy and mental clarity, better weight management, improved blood sugar control, reduced inflammation, and improved longevity and anti-aging effects.

Improved Hormone Balance

Hormone balance is crucial for women's health, as imbalances can lead to a range of issues, from menstrual irregularities to mood disorders. Intermittent fasting has been shown to improve hormone balance by reducing insulin levels and increasing growth hormone levels.

Insulin is a hormone that regulates blood sugar levels, and high insulin levels can lead to insulin resistance and increased risk of chronic diseases such as diabetes and heart disease. Intermittent fasting can help to reduce insulin levels and improve insulin sensitivity, which can lead to better blood sugar control and reduced inflammation.

Growth hormone is another hormone that plays a key role in women's health, as it promotes muscle growth and repair, and improves bone density. Intermittent fasting has been shown to increase growth hormone levels, which can help to improve muscle growth and repair, and reduce the risk of osteoporosis.

Increased Energy and Mental Clarity

Many women report increased energy and mental clarity when they adopt intermittent fasting. This may be due to the fact that fasting can improve mitochondrial function, which is the process by which cells produce energy. Fasting can also improve brain function by increasing the production of brain-derived neurotrophic factor (BDNF), a protein that is important for learning and memory.

Better Weight Management

Weight management is a concern for many women, and intermittent fasting can be an effective tool for weight loss and weight management. By creating a calorie deficit and inducing a state of ketosis, intermittent fasting can lead to increased fat burning and improved metabolic health.

Intermittent fasting has also been shown to reduce appetite and increase feelings of fullness, which can help women to consume fewer calories overall. This can lead to sustainable weight loss and improved weight management over time.

Improved Blood Sugar Control

Blood sugar control is important for women's health, as high blood sugar levels can lead to insulin resistance and increased risk of chronic diseases. Intermittent fasting can help to improve blood sugar control by reducing insulin levels and increasing insulin sensitivity.

Reduced Inflammation

Inflammation is a key driver of many chronic diseases, and reducing inflammation is crucial for maintaining optimal health and wellbeing. Intermittent fasting has been shown to reduce inflammation by improving insulin sensitivity and reducing oxidative stress.

Improved Longevity and Anti-Aging Effects

Intermittent fasting has been shown to improve longevity and have anti-aging effects, which may be due to its ability to improve mitochondrial function, reduce inflammation, and improve hormone balance. Intermittent fasting has been shown to increase lifespan and improve markers of aging in animal studies, and it may have similar effects in humans.

Overall, intermittent fasting can provide a range of benefits for women, from improved hormone balance to increased energy and mental clarity, better weight management, improved blood sugar control, reduced inflammation, and improved longevity and anti-aging effects. By adopting a thoughtful and intentional approach to intermittent fasting, women can harness the power of this eating strategy to achieve optimal health and wellbeing. However, it is important to note that intermittent fasting may not be appropriate for all women, particularly those who are pregnant or breastfeeding, have a history of disordered eating or have underlying health conditions. It is always important to consult with a healthcare professional before starting any new dietary or lifestyle changes.

Tips for Women Practicing Intermittent Fasting

While intermittent fasting can provide many benefits for women, it is important to approach it in a thoughtful and intentional way to ensure optimal results. Here are some tips for women practicing intermittent fasting:

- Start slow and gradually increase fasting duration: If you are new to intermittent fasting, it is important to start slow and gradually increase the duration of your fasts. Begin with a 12-hour fast and gradually increase the duration to 16 or 18 hours as your body adapts.

- Choose the right type of intermittent fasting: There are several types of intermittent fasting, and it is important to choose the right one for your body and lifestyle. Consider factors such as your work schedule, exercise routine, and any underlying health conditions when choosing an intermittent fasting plan.

- Stay hydrated: It is important to stay hydrated during your fasting periods. Drink plenty of water, herbal tea, or other non-caloric beverages to support your body's needs.

- Focus on nutrient-dense meals: When you break your fast, focus on consuming nutrient-dense meals that provide a balance of macronutrients and micronutrients. This can help to support your body's needs and prevent cravings or overeating.

- Listen to your body: It is important to listen to your body and adjust your fasting routine as needed. If you feel overly fatigued, lightheaded, or experience any other adverse symptoms, it may be time to adjust your fasting routine or consult with a healthcare professional.

Conclusion

Intermittent fasting can provide many benefits for women, from improved hormone balance to increased energy and mental clarity, better weight management, improved blood sugar control, reduced inflammation, and improved longevity and anti-aging effects. By adopting a thoughtful and intentional approach to intermittent fasting, women can harness the power of this eating strategy to achieve optimal health and wellbeing. However, it is important to approach intermittent fasting in a safe and sustainable way, and to consult with a healthcare professional before starting any new dietary or lifestyle changes. With the right approach, intermittent fasting can be a powerful tool for women's health and wellbeing.

Chapter 3

How to Get Started with Intermittent Fasting

Intermittent fasting is an eating strategy that has gained popularity in recent years for its potential health benefits. If you're interested in trying intermittent fasting, it can be helpful to have a plan in place to help you get started. In this chapter, we'll discuss how to assess your current diet and lifestyle, choose the right intermittent fasting plan for you, set realistic goals, and provide tips and strategies for making intermittent fasting easier.

Assessing Your Current Diet and Lifestyle

Before starting intermittent fasting, it is important to assess your current diet and lifestyle to ensure that you are approaching this eating strategy in a safe and sustainable way. Here are some key factors to consider when assessing your current diet and lifestyle:

- Current eating habits: Take a close look at your current eating habits. Do you tend to eat throughout the day or consume large meals in the evening? Understanding your current eating habits can help you choose the right intermittent fasting plan for you.

- Exercise routine: Consider your current exercise routine. Do you engage in regular physical activity? This can impact your fasting schedule and the type of fasting plan you choose.

- Sleep patterns: Adequate sleep is essential for overall health and wellbeing. Consider your current sleep patterns and aim to prioritize adequate rest as you begin your intermittent fasting journey.

- Underlying health conditions: If you have any underlying health conditions, it is important to consult with a healthcare professional before starting intermittent fasting to ensure that it is safe and appropriate for you.

Choosing the Right Intermittent Fasting Plan for You
There are several types of intermittent fasting, and it is important to choose the right one for your body and lifestyle. Here are some of the most common types of intermittent fasting:

- Time-restricted feeding: Time-restricted feeding involves limiting your eating to a specific window of time each day, typically 8-10 hours. This can be a good option for beginners or those with a busy schedule.

- Alternate day fasting: Alternate day fasting involves fasting every other day or consuming very low calorie meals on fasting days. This can be a more challenging fasting plan, but may provide greater benefits for weight loss and other health markers.

- 5:2 fasting: 5:2 fasting involves eating normally for five days of the week and consuming only 500-600 calories on two non-consecutive days of the week. This can be a more flexible fasting plan that allows for more varied eating throughout the week.

- 24-hour fasting: 24-hour fasting involves fasting for a full 24 hours once or twice a week. This can be a more challenging fasting plan, but may provide greater benefits for weight loss and other health markers.

When choosing an intermittent fasting plan, consider your current eating habits, exercise routine, and underlying health conditions. It is also important to choose a plan that is sustainable and realistic for your lifestyle.

Setting Realistic Goals

As with any lifestyle change, it is important to set realistic goals for your intermittent fasting journey. Here are some tips for setting realistic goals:

- Start small: If you're new to intermittent fasting, it can be helpful to start with a shorter fasting window and gradually increase the duration as your body adapts.

- Focus on health goals: While weight loss is a common goal of intermittent fasting, it is important to focus on overall health and wellbeing as well. Consider setting goals related to improved energy, mental clarity, or other health markers.

- Be patient: Intermittent fasting is not a quick fix, and it can take time to see results. Be patient with yourself and trust the process.

Tips and Strategies for Making Intermittent Fasting Easier

Intermittent fasting can be challenging, especially for beginners. However, with the right mindset and some helpful strategies, it can become a natural part of your daily routine. Here are some tips to make the transition to intermittent fasting easier:

- Start with a shorter fasting period: If you're new to intermittent fasting, you may want to start with a shorter fasting period, such as 12 hours. As you get used to it, you can gradually increase the duration.

- Stay hydrated: Drinking plenty of water is essential during fasting periods. It can help you stay full, reduce hunger pangs, and flush out toxins from your body.

- Distract yourself: Keeping busy and engaged in other activities can help take your mind off food and make fasting periods easier. Consider going for a walk, reading a book, or practicing meditation.

- Plan your meals: Planning your meals ahead of time can help you avoid the temptation to break your fast. Have healthy, balanced meals ready for when you break your fast to ensure you're getting all the nutrients you need.

- Don't overeat during your feeding window: It can be tempting to indulge in unhealthy foods during your feeding window, but doing so can negate the benefits of intermittent fasting. Stick to healthy, whole foods and avoid overeating.

Conclusion

Intermittent fasting is a powerful tool for improving health and wellbeing. For women, it can be particularly beneficial due to its ability to balance hormones, improve energy levels, promote weight loss, regulate blood sugar, reduce inflammation, and promote longevity. However, it's essential to approach intermittent fasting with caution and ensure you're choosing the right plan for your body and lifestyle. With patience, dedication, and the right mindset, you can

22

make intermittent fasting a sustainable part of your healthy lifestyle.

Chapter 4

Overcoming Common Challenges with Intermittent Fasting

Intermittent fasting can offer numerous benefits for women, but it's not always easy to stick to the plan. Many women may face common challenges that can make it difficult to stay on track with their fasting goals. In this chapter, we'll discuss some of the most common challenges women face with intermittent fasting and provide tips for overcoming them.

Hunger and Cravings

One of the most significant challenges with intermittent fasting is dealing with hunger and cravings. When you're used to eating three meals a day plus snacks, cutting back to a restricted eating window can be challenging at first. However, there are several strategies you can use to manage hunger and cravings during your fasting periods.

- Drink plenty of water: Staying hydrated can help reduce hunger and cravings. Aim to drink at least 8-10 glasses of water per day, and consider adding lemon or lime for flavor.

- Stay busy: Keeping busy can help take your mind off of food. Try doing a puzzle, going for a walk, or engaging in a hobby during your fasting periods.

- Drink tea or coffee: Sipping on herbal tea or black coffee can help suppress your appetite and keep you feeling full.

- Choose nutrient-dense foods: When you do eat during your feeding window, choose foods that are high in protein and fiber. These foods will keep you feeling full and satisfied for longer.

Social Situations and Dining Out

Social situations and dining out can be challenging when you're following an intermittent fasting plan. However, with a little planning, you can still enjoy these activities while staying on track with your fasting goals.

- Plan ahead: Check the menu before you go out to eat and choose healthy options that fit within your feeding window.

- Eat a small snack beforehand: Eating a small, nutrient-dense snack before going out can help curb your appetite and prevent overeating.

- Communicate with others: Let your friends and family know about your fasting plan so they can support you and help you stick to your goals.

Balancing Intermittent Fasting with Exercise

Exercise is an essential component of a healthy lifestyle, but it can be challenging to balance with intermittent fasting. Many women may experience low energy levels during fasting periods, making exercise more difficult. However, there are several strategies you can use to maintain your fitness routine while still following your fasting plan.

- Choose the right time to exercise: Try scheduling your workouts during your feeding window to ensure you have enough energy to power through your workout.

- Start slow: If you're new to exercise, start with low-intensity workouts and gradually build up your stamina over time.

- Stay hydrated: Drinking plenty of water before, during, and after exercise can help you maintain energy levels and prevent dehydration.

Managing Menstruation and Hormonal Changes

Many women experience hormonal changes throughout their menstrual cycle, which can affect energy levels and appetite. It's important to be mindful of these changes when following an intermittent fasting plan and make adjustments as needed.

- Listen to your body: If you're feeling particularly hungry or fatigued during your menstrual cycle, it's okay to adjust your fasting schedule or extend your feeding window.

- Eat nutrient-dense foods: During menstruation, it's essential to consume nutrient-dense foods to support energy levels and overall health.

- Consider a modified plan: Some women may find it helpful to modify their intermittent fasting plan during their menstrual cycle. For example, they may choose to fast for shorter periods or opt for a different fasting schedule altogether.

Conclusion

While intermittent fasting can offer numerous health benefits for women, there are also challenges that must be addressed. By implementing strategies to overcome hunger and cravings, navigating social situations and dining out, balancing fasting with exercise, and managing hormonal changes, women can successfully incorporate intermittent fasting into their lives and reap the benefits of this powerful health tool.

Chapter 5

Maximizing the Benefits of Intermittent Fasting

Intermittent fasting is an effective way to improve overall health and wellness, but it is important to note that it is not a magic bullet. To truly maximize the benefits of intermittent fasting, it is essential to adopt healthy lifestyle habits in addition to practicing intermittent fasting. In this chapter, we will explore the various ways to complement and enhance intermittent fasting for optimal health and wellness.

The Importance of a Balanced and Nutritious Diet

Intermittent fasting is not a license to indulge in unhealthy eating habits during the eating window. To maximize the benefits of intermittent fasting, it is crucial to consume a balanced and nutritious diet. This means eating plenty of vegetables, fruits, whole grains, and lean proteins. It is also important to limit or avoid processed foods, refined carbohydrates, and added sugars, which can lead to inflammation and other health issues.

Incorporating Exercise and Movement

While intermittent fasting can help with weight loss and improve overall health, incorporating exercise and movement can further enhance these benefits. Exercise can help build muscle, increase bone density, improve cardiovascular health, and boost metabolism. It is important to note that exercise does not have to be high-intensity or strenuous; even low-impact activities like walking or yoga can provide significant health benefits.

Managing Stress and Getting Enough Sleep

Stress and lack of sleep can have a negative impact on overall health and wellness. Chronic stress can lead to inflammation, weakened immune function, and increased risk of chronic diseases. Meanwhile, inadequate sleep can affect hormone regulation, metabolism, and cognitive function. Therefore, it is crucial to prioritize stress management techniques like meditation, deep breathing, or spending time in nature, as well as ensuring adequate sleep.

Supplements and Other Tools for Enhancing Intermittent Fasting

While a balanced and nutritious diet, exercise, stress management, and sleep are essential for maximizing the benefits of intermittent fasting, some supplements and other tools can also help. These include:

- Probiotics: These supplements can help support gut health, improve digestion, and boost the immune system.

- Omega-3 fatty acids: Found in fatty fish, nuts, and seeds, omega-3 fatty acids can help reduce inflammation and support heart health.

- Fiber: Eating plenty of fiber can help regulate digestion, promote feelings of fullness, and support a healthy gut microbiome.

- Water: Staying hydrated is crucial for overall health and can help reduce feelings of hunger during fasting periods.

- Intermittent fasting apps: There are many apps available that can help track fasting periods and provide guidance and support for beginners.

- Mindful eating practices: Mindful eating techniques like chewing slowly, savoring flavors, and paying attention to hunger and fullness signals can help improve digestion and reduce overeating during the eating window.

Conclusion

Intermittent fasting is a powerful tool for improving overall health and wellness. By adopting a healthy and balanced diet, incorporating exercise and movement, managing stress, and getting adequate sleep, individuals can maximize the benefits of intermittent fasting. Additionally, supplements and other tools can provide added support for optimal health and wellness. With dedication, patience, and perseverance, anyone can successfully incorporate intermittent fasting into their lifestyle and achieve their health and wellness goals.

Chapter 6

Long-Term Success with Intermittent Fasting

While intermittent fasting can provide numerous benefits for women in terms of weight management, hormone balance, energy, and overall health, it's important to approach it as a long-term lifestyle change rather than a quick fix. In this chapter, we'll discuss how to create healthy habits and lifestyle changes that support sustainable intermittent fasting, as well as how to monitor your progress and make adjustments along the way. We'll also explore how to balance intermittent fasting with other health goals and priorities.

Creating Healthy Habits and Lifestyle Changes

One of the keys to long-term success with intermittent fasting is creating healthy habits and lifestyle changes that support your fasting routine. This includes making changes to your diet, exercise routine, sleep habits, and stress management techniques.

- Diet: It's important to eat a balanced and nutritious diet to support your intermittent fasting routine. This means focusing on whole, nutrient-dense foods like fruits, vegetables, lean proteins, and healthy fats. It's also important to stay hydrated and avoid excessive amounts of sugar, processed foods, and alcohol.

- Exercise: Regular exercise can help support weight loss and improve overall health, but it's important to balance your exercise routine with your intermittent fasting schedule. If you're doing longer fasts, you may want to avoid high-intensity workouts during your fasting period, as this can put stress on your body. Instead, focus on low to moderate intensity activities like walking, yoga, or light weight lifting.

- Sleep: Getting enough sleep is crucial for overall health and well-being, but it's especially important when you're fasting. Lack of sleep can increase feelings of hunger and lead to overeating, making it harder to stick to your fasting routine. Aim for 7-8 hours of sleep per night and try to establish a consistent sleep schedule.

- Stress Management: Stress can interfere with your fasting routine and overall health. Finding effective ways to manage stress, such as meditation, yoga, or deep breathing exercises, can help support your fasting routine and improve your overall well-being.

Monitoring Your Progress and Making Adjustments
As you begin your intermittent fasting journey, it's important to track your progress and make adjustments as needed. This can help you stay on track with your goals and ensure that you're getting the most out of your fasting routine.

One way to monitor your progress is to keep a food diary or use a tracking app to log your meals, fasting periods, and any symptoms or changes you experience. This can help you identify patterns and make adjustments as needed, such as adjusting your fasting schedule or tweaking your diet.

Another important aspect of monitoring your progress is getting regular check-ups with your healthcare provider. This can help identify any underlying health issues that may be impacting your ability to fast or achieve your goals.

Finally, it's important to be flexible and open to making adjustments to your fasting routine as needed. What works for one person may not work for another, so it's important to listen to your body and make changes that support your individual needs and goals.

Balancing Intermittent Fasting with Other Health Goals and Priorities
While intermittent fasting can be an effective tool for weight management and overall health, it's important to balance it with other health goals and priorities. This

includes things like maintaining a healthy social life, taking care of your mental health, and addressing any underlying health issues.

- Social Life: Social situations can be challenging when you're fasting, but it's important to maintain a healthy social life. You can still enjoy meals and activities with friends and family while fasting, but you may need to adjust your schedule or approach to accommodate your fasting routine.

- Mental Health: Intermittent fasting has also been found to have a positive impact on mental health. Studies have shown that intermittent fasting may help improve mood, reduce anxiety, and even improve cognitive function. One theory is that this may be due to the increase in brain-derived neurotrophic factor (BDNF), a protein that plays a role in nerve cell growth and development.

In addition, intermittent fasting may help reduce inflammation, which has been linked to depression and other mental health disorders. By reducing inflammation, intermittent fasting may help improve overall brain health and reduce the risk of mental health issues.

Safety Considerations

Intermittent fasting can be a safe and effective way to improve health and wellbeing, but it is important to approach it with caution, especially for women. While some studies have shown that intermittent fasting can be beneficial for women, others have suggested that it may have negative effects on reproductive health and hormones.

It is important to talk to a healthcare provider before starting an intermittent fasting regimen, especially if you have any underlying health conditions or are taking any medications. Pregnant or breastfeeding women, as well as women with a history of disordered eating, should not attempt intermittent fasting without medical supervision.

Additionally, it is important to listen to your body and be mindful of any changes in your physical or mental health while fasting. If you experience any adverse effects, such as dizziness, headaches, or weakness, it is important to stop fasting and seek medical attention if necessary.

Conclusion

Intermittent fasting is a powerful tool that can help women improve their overall health and wellbeing. By reducing inflammation, improving hormone balance, and promoting weight loss, intermittent fasting can have a wide range of benefits for women of all ages and fitness levels.

However, it is important to approach intermittent fasting with caution and to talk to a healthcare provider before starting a fasting regimen. By setting realistic goals, making small changes to your diet and lifestyle, and incorporating other healthy habits, such as exercise and stress management, you can maximize the benefits of intermittent fasting and achieve long-term success.

Chapter 7

Conclusion

The Power of Intermittent Fasting for Women: Achieving Optimal Health and Fitness

Intermittent fasting is a powerful tool for women looking to improve their overall health and fitness. By incorporating periods of calorie restriction and intentional eating, women can benefit from improved hormone balance, increased energy and mental clarity, better weight management, improved blood sugar control, reduced inflammation, and improved longevity and anti-aging effects.

It's important to note that intermittent fasting is not a one-size-fits-all approach, and women should carefully assess their current diet and lifestyle before starting a fasting protocol. It's also essential to choose the right fasting plan, set realistic goals, and implement strategies to make fasting easier.

While fasting can be challenging at times, it's important to remember that hunger and cravings are normal and can be managed with the right mindset and tools. Social situations and exercise should also be taken into consideration when implementing a fasting plan.

To maximize the benefits of intermittent fasting, women should focus on a balanced and nutritious diet, incorporate regular exercise and movement, manage stress and prioritize adequate sleep, and consider supplements and other tools to enhance their fasting experience.

Long-term success with intermittent fasting requires creating healthy habits and lifestyle changes, monitoring progress, and making adjustments as necessary. Women should also balance their fasting goals with other health priorities and strive for a holistic approach to their health and wellness.

Final Thoughts and Actionable Steps

Intermittent fasting can be a powerful tool for women looking to improve their health and fitness, but it's important to approach fasting with a mindful and intentional mindset. By carefully assessing your current diet and lifestyle, choosing the right fasting plan, and implementing strategies to make fasting easier, you can successfully incorporate fasting into your routine.

Remember that fasting can be challenging at times, but hunger and cravings are normal and can be managed with the right mindset and tools. Focus on a balanced and nutritious diet, regular exercise and movement, managing stress and prioritizing adequate sleep, and considering supplements and other tools to enhance your fasting experience.

Long-term success with intermittent fasting requires creating healthy habits and lifestyle changes, monitoring progress, and making adjustments as necessary. Remember to balance your fasting goals with other health priorities and strive for a holistic approach to your health and wellness.

In conclusion, the power of intermittent fasting for women is undeniable, and with the right approach, women can achieve optimal health and fitness. Start today by assessing your current diet and lifestyle, choosing the right fasting plan, and implementing strategies to make fasting easier. Here's to your health and success on your intermittent fasting journey!